How To Lose Weight Fast In A Healthy And Sustainable Way

The Best Diet Plan For Safe Weight Loss

DR. ADAM COLTON

Published by BizMove
www.bizmove.com

<u>Important Disclaimer</u>
Please See This Before You Start Reading The Book

All the content found in this book was created for informational purposes only. The Content is not intended to be a substitute for professional medical advice, diagnosis, or treatment. Always seek the advice of your physician or other qualified health provider with any questions you may have regarding a medical condition. Never disregard professional medical advice or delay in seeking it because of something you have read in this book.

ISBN: 1977934773

ISBN-13: 978-1977934772

Table of Contents

1. How This Book Can Help You Lose Weight

The secret to success in a diet is making changes and sticking with them. in this book you'll learn exactly how to develop a weight loss strategy that really get results. It is simple, it is easy and it produces fast results.

First of all, this diet plan works fast. It literally burns off fat by the hour. If you go on this diet in the morning you will lose weight before lunch. You lose weight faster on this diet than if you ran 7 miles every day. You'll be able to measure the difference in your waistline in 24 to 36 hours. I think this is the fastest safe diet in the world. If you find a diet that works faster I will buy it from you and gladly pay good money for it.

Healthy & Safe

This is not just a weight-loss diet. It's a healthy diet also. It is safe. It is probably much safer than the way you are right now. Don't ever take a chance with your health. It's not worth it. Besides it is not necessary. You can lose weight fast on this diet plus get healthier every day you stay on it.

Automatic Weight Loss

Right after you go on the diet you start to lose weight automatically. You don't have to think about it all the time. You would probably forget you're on a diet if you weren't losing weight so fast.

As you can tell by now I've come up with something pretty good. I think this diet is the best way to lose weight I have ever heard about. You lose weight very fast. You can eat out as often as you like. Your health will improve and your energy will increase. Except for when you weigh yourself you'll probably forget you're on a diet.

In short, this diet is fast, safe and simple.

This diet plan is different from any other. it has a different plan of attack. This diet forces you to form a very new habit. This new habit is pleasurable and fun. This habit makes it possible to stay on any diet for life without ever feeling deprived. This new habit makes everything easy. It is so simple you will wonder why you never thought of it yourself.

It is simple to apply yet highly effective **Healthy Weight Loss Plan**. In addition to helping you feel and look better, reaching a healthier body weight is good for your overall health and well being. If you are overweight or obese, you have a greater risk of developing many diseases including type 2 diabetes, heart disease, and some types of cancer.

The secret to success is making changes and sticking with them. This plan is comprised of three essential components:

First - Find out What You Eat and Drink. This is a key step in managing your weight.

Next - Find out What to Eat and Drink. Get a personalized Daily Food Plan - just for you - to help guide your food choices.

Then - Make Better Choices. Everyone is different. Compare what you eat and drink to what you should eat and drink. The ideas and tips in this section can help you make better choices, which can have a lasting impact on your body weight over time.

2. Learn What You Currently Eat and Drink

Did you know that:

The #1 source of calories in the American diet is desserts - like cakes and cookies?

Americans get more calories from sugary drinks than any other beverage choice?

Identifying what you are eating and drinking now will help you see where you can make better choices in the future.

If you want to make changes to improve the way you eat and your body weight, the first step is to identify what you do now. This includes becoming more aware of:

What and how much you eat and drink

How physically active you are

Your body weight

People who are most successful at losing weight and keeping it off track their intake regularly. Tracking physical activity and body weight can also help you reach your weight goals.

Here's how to identify what you eat and drink:

Write down what and how_much you eat and drink. Find a way that works for you. Use a journal, log your intake on your calendar, keep track on your phone, or use an online

tool like the SuperTracker
(https://www.supertracker.usda.gov/).

Start by identifying what you've already eaten today. Be sure to include how much as well as what you ate. Don't forget to include drinks, sauces, spreads, and sides. It all counts.

In addition, write down the physical activities you do, and how long you spend doing each one. Log each activity that you do for at least 10 minutes at a time. Every bit adds up. Use the SuperTracker (https://www.supertracker.usda.gov/), a journal, or mark a calendar.

Once you've identified what you are doing now, keep it up! Tracking what and how much you eat and drink, your body weight, and your physical activity can help you manage your body weight over the long term.

Concerned about identifying what you eat and drink? Here are some common "stumbling blocks" and ideas to help you overcome these barriers:

"I'm interested in using an online tool, but I don't have internet access every day": If you don't have regular access to a computer, you can begin by simply writing down what, when, and how much you eat in a journal. Just writing down what you eat and drink helps you become more aware.

When you are able to access a computer, you can enter

several days of intake into the SuperTracker (https://www.supertracker.usda.gov/) at once.

"It takes a lot of time to track my intake"*:* The fact is that tracking works. Find a way that you can track your intake that works for you – whether it be writing what and how much you eat and drink in a journal, your day planner, or your calendar. With the SuperTracker (https://www.supertracker.usda.gov/), you can develop lists of your favorite foods that can help you enter your intake more quickly.

"By the time I get to a computer, I've forgotten what I ate"*:* For tracking to work, it needs to be complete. If necessary, carry a food journal or log your intake on your smart phone. Logging what you eat immediately will help your tracking to be more accurate.

"I can identify what I ate, but have no idea of how to figure out how much I ate": Measure out foods you regularly eat (such as a bowl of cereal) once or twice, to get a sense of how big your typical portion is. Also measure out what 1/2 or 1 cup portion size looks like to help you estimate how much you eat.

Check the serving size information on the Nutrition Facts label (https://www.nhlbi.nih.gov/health/educational/wecan/eat -right/nutrition-facts.htm) of packaged foods. It describes what the "standard" serving size is, and how many are in the package.

3. What To Eat and Drink

Use the Daily Food Plans
(https://www.choosemyplate.gov/MyPlate-Daily-
Checklist) to help you choose foods and beverages that
meet your nutrient needs while staying within your calorie
limits. Think of your Food Plan as a roadmap to guide you
on the path to a healthier weight. Learn how much you
need to eat each day from the 5 food groups. You can also
find out your total calorie limit and your limit for empty
calories (calories from solid fats and added sugars) with
your Daily Food Plan
(https://www.choosemyplate.gov/MyPlate-Daily-
Checklist).

Your Food Plan is not a quick weight loss program. It's a
way to eat for health and well being. If you stick with the
Plan over time, you should gradually move toward a
healthier weight.

Here's How to Find Out What to Eat and Drink:

Enter your age, sex, height, weight, and activity level in the
Daily Food Plan entry box
(https://www.choosemyplate.gov/MyPlate-Daily-
Checklist-input).

If you are not within your healthy weight range, the Plan
lets you choose an option to gradually move to a healthier
weight. This option provides 200 to 400 calories less per
day than the average calorie needs to maintain your weight.

Once you've entered your information and picked the "move toward a healthier weight" option, you will get a plan with your calorie limits and the amounts to eat and drink from each food group every day. Following this plan can help you gradually lose weight. You can print your plan for future quick access.

Concerned about following a Food Plan? Here are some common "stumbling blocks" and ideas to help you overcome these barriers:

"I get frustrated because I don't see results fast enough": Most people gain weight slowly over time, even years. Chances are that you gained weight slowly over time, and it will take time to lose your excess body weight. You will be more successful at keeping weight off if you lose it gradually and not over a short period of time.

You don't have to reach a healthy body weight to start experiencing improvements in health. Losing 5% to 10% of your current body weight can have health benefits.

It's also important to track your success at making changes. For example, if your goal is to go on a 15-minute walk each day during your lunch break, then consider accomplishing this goal as a success. Results on the scale may be more gradual, but you are still making positive changes.

"I don't have the will power to stick to a plan": You don't have to change everything you do all at once. Try making one change at a time, like decreasing portion sizes, then after that has become routine, make more changes. It can also help if you have friends or family who are making changes with you. On the SuperTracker, you can also sign up for regular text messages to keep you motivated in "My Coach Center."

"Can't I just skip meals to lose weight?": It's important to eat enough, but not too much. Skipping meals isn't the answer for long term success at managing your weight. The goal is to pick the best food and beverage options in the right amounts. Your Daily Food Plan shows you what and how much to eat and drink from each food group. Stick to your Plan instead of skipping meals.

"The Daily Food Plan looks like too much food – I'll never lose weight if I eat all of this": An important part of the Plan is to make nutrient-dense choices in each food group. This means choosing foods and beverages with little or no solid fats and added sugars. Solid fats and added sugars make up about 35% of most Americans' calorie intake. If you choose foods without them, you can eat a lot, feel full, and still lose weight gradually.

4. How to Construct Your Weight Loss Strategy

When you compare what you eat to your Daily Food Plan (https://www.choosemyplate.gov/MyPlate-Daily-Checklist), is there room for improvement? For example, do you eat many sweets or fried foods? Do you drink sugary drinks regularly? Do you eat too few vegetables or whole grains? Does eating out make it difficult to stay on track?

Everyone is different. Think about what you eat and drink. How can you make better choices? How can you be more active? The SuperTracker can help you identify changes you should make.

Now, you can construct your weight loss plan by utilizing the below strategies. Making these changes and sticking with them can help you manage your body weight.

* Eat the Right Amount of Calories for You

* Decrease Portion Sizes

* Eat Fewer Empty Calories

* Focus on Foods You Need

* When Eating Out, Make Better Choices

* Cook More Often at Home

* Increase Physical Activity

* Decrease Television and Computer Time

In the following chapter we will discuss each of these strategies.

---

5. Eat the Right Amount of Calories for You

Everyone has a personal calorie limit. Staying within yours can help you get to or maintain a healthy weight. Reaching a healthier weight is a balancing act. The secret is learning how to balance your "energy in" and "energy out" over the long run. "Energy in" is the calories from foods and beverages you have each day. "Energy out" is the calories you burn for basic body functions and physical activity.

A balancing act: Where is your energy balance?

Maintaining weight — Your weight will stay the same when the calories you eat and drink equal the calories you burn.

Losing weight — You will lose weight when the calories you eat and drink are less than the calories you burn.

Gaining weight — You will gain weight when the calories you eat and drink are greater than the calories you burn.

The current high rates of overweight and obesity in the United States mean that many people are taking in more calories than they burn.

Get started eating the right amount of calories for you:

Get your personal daily calorie limit. Enter your age, sex, height, weight, and activity level in the Daily Food Plan entry box (https://www.choosemyplate.gov/MyPlate-Daily-Checklist-input). If you are not within your healthy weight range, pick the "move toward a healthier weight" option. This option provides 200 to 400 calories less per day than the average calorie needs to maintain your weight. Your Daily Food Plan will include a total calorie limit.

Keep your calorie limit in mind when deciding what to eat and drink. For example, if your calorie limit is 1,800 calories per day, think about how those calories can be split up among meals, snacks, and beverages over the course of a day.It doesn't have to be the same each day. If you eat a larger lunch, think about eating a smaller meal at dinner.

Compare food and beverage options and think about how they fit within your calorie limit. For example, a snack with 200 calories may be a better option than another with 500 calories. Use your daily calorie limit to help you decide which foods and drinks to choose.

For a healthier you, use the Nutrition Facts label to make smart food choices quickly and easily. Check the label of similar products for calories, and choose the food with fewer calories. Be sure to look at the serving size and how many servings you are actually consuming, as well. If you eat twice the serving size, you double the calories. When eating out, calorie information may be available on menus, in a pamphlet, or online. You can also find calorie information about a specific food using Food-a-pedia (https://www.supertracker.usda.gov/foodapedia.aspx).

Concerned about being able to eat the right amount of calories? Here are some common "stumbling blocks" and ideas to help you overcome these barriers:

"I don't understand calories": need while staying within your calorie limits. Use your Daily Food Plan to determine how much you should eat from each of the 5 food groups.

"I don't have time to count calories": People who are successful at managing their weight have found ways to keep track of how much they eat in a day, even if they don't count every calorie. Most people eat the same general types of food on a regular basis. Take some time up front to compare calorie labels, and over time, you will learn which options are the better choices.

Also, if you Focus on Foods You Need (see below) and Eat Fewer Empty Calories (see below) you will be a big step closer to eating the right amount of calories for you.

"I don't have time to count calories": People who are successful at managing their weight have found ways to keep track of how much they eat in a day, even if they don't count every calorie. Most people eat the same general types of food on a regular basis. Take some time up front to compare calorie labels, and over time, you will learn which options are the better choices.

"I have no idea how many calories I am supposed to eat to manage my weight": Your calorie needs depend on a number of factors including: your height, weight, and physical activity level. You can get your personal daily calorie limit with your Daily Food Plan (https://www.choosemyplate.gov/MyPlate-Daily-Checklist). Try to stay at (or a little below) this number each day. Taking in more calories (even just 100 calories more each day) can result in gradual weight gain over time.

The calories in your Daily Food Plan are averages. For best results, track your body weight over time. If you are gaining weight, or not losing at all, decrease your calorie intake (or increase your physical activity).

6. Decrease Portion Sizes

The amount you eat or drink plays an important role in your energy balance strategy. Most people eat and drink more when served larger portions. Choosing smaller portions can help you lose weight and keep it off.

Portions have increased over time. You may be eating more than you realize. Some common food portions can equal the amount that is recommended for the whole day. For example, on a 1600 calorie Daily Food Plan, 5 ounces a day of grains are suggested. Some bagels weigh up to 5 ounces - the entire day's allotment of grains!

Your Daily Food Plan (https://www.choosemyplate.gov/MyPlate-Daily-Checklist) helps you manage your daily intake by recommending the amount of food you need from each food group.

Your portions at each meal do not need to be any specific amount-but to stay within your energy needs, the total amount you eat *each day* should match the total amount recommended for each group. For example, 1 regular slice of bread counts as 1 ounce of grains. This doesn't mean that you have to eat a sandwich with one piece of bread. It just means that if you eat two slices, you should count them both toward your total grain intake for the day.

Get started eating smaller portions:

Figure out how big your portions really are: Measure how much the bowls, glasses, cups, and plates you usually use hold. Pour your breakfast cereal into your regular bowl. Then, pour it into a measuring cup. How many cups of cereal do you eat each day?

Measure a fixed amount of some foods and drinks to see what they look like in your glasses and plates. For example, measure 1 cup of juice to see what 1 cup of liquid looks like in your favorite glass. To see what 1 cup, ½ cup, or 1 ounce of some different foods looks like, Prepare, serve, and eat smaller portions of food. Start by portioning out small amounts to eat and drink. Only go back for more if you are still hungry.

Pay attention to feelings of hunger. Stop eating when you are satisfied, not full. If there is still food on your plate or on the table, put it away (or throw it out). Repeat the phrase "a moment on the lips, a year on the hips" as you do this.

A simple trick to help you eat less is to use a smaller plate, bowl, or glass. One cup of food on a small plate looks like more than the same cup of food on a large plate.

It is important to think about portion sizes when eating out. Order a smaller size option, when it's available. Manage larger portions by sharing or taking home part of your meal. When Eating Out, Make Better Choices (see below) has lots of tips to help you eat only the amount you need when eating out.

If you tend to overeat, be aware of the time of day, place, and your mood while eating so you can better control the amount you eat. Some people overeat when stressed or upset. Try walking instead of eating, or snack on a healthier option. For example, instead of eating a bag of chips, crunch on some celery, or instead of eating a bowl of ice cream, enjoy a low-fat yogurt with fresh blueberries. Making healthier choices is better for your weight and can also help you feel better.

Concerned about eating smaller portion sizes? Here are some common "stumbling blocks" and ideas to help you overcome these barriers:

"I don't have time to measure out my foods all the time": Being successful at decreasing portion sizes doesn't mean that you have to measure every meal or snack you eat. Once you've taken the time to measure out a few examples, you will be able to estimate portion sizes better. Plus, just eating or drinking less than you normally would means you are decreasing your portion sizes.

"My Daily Food Plan tells me to eat more of some things but also to decrease portion sizes. I don't understand if I should eat more or less": The recommendation to decrease portion sizes is particularly important for high calorie foods or for foods with a lot of empty calories, such as cakes, cookies, sugary drinks, and pizza. It is important to Focus on Foods You Need. For example, eat a large portion of steamed broccoli (but with only a very small amount of butter or cheese sauce, if any).

"I like to eat a big burger every once in a while. Are there other ways to eat less?": In general, it is a good rule to eat and drink smaller portions. You can occasionally eat or drink foods in larger portions, but not as part of your daily diet. Make that big burger a "once-in-a-while" special treat, and on most days choose the smaller options.

"I was always told to clean my plate.": Resign from the "clean your plate" club **now**. Stop eating when you are satisfied, not when your plate is empty. Start your meal by only eating half of what's on your plate. Stop for a moment and decide if you really want to eat more. Don't forget that you can save some leftovers for another meal or snack. Nothing has to go to waste, and the food will taste better when you are hungry again!

7. Eat Fewer Empty Calories

A great way to help you manage your body weight is to eat fewer empty calories. Empty calories are calories from solid fats, added sugars, or both.

Many empty calories that Americans eat come from foods and beverages that provide calories but few nutrients--such as desserts, sodas, and candies. Added sugars and fats load these choices with extra calories you don't need.

Some foods and beverages provide essential nutrients, but may also contain some empty calories. For example, a cup of whole milk contains about 150 calories, with over 60 of them empty calories from fat. Fat-free milk has the same amount of calcium and other nutrients as whole milk, but with less than 90 calories and no fat or empty calories.

Regardless of your weight status, empty calories should not be a major part of the diet. For most people, no more than 15% of calories should come from solid fats and added sugars. However, about 35% of the calories Americans typically eat and drink are empty calories. This means that many people choose foods and drinks with TOO MUCH solid fats and added sugars.

Get Started Eating Fewer Empty Calories:

Here are three ways to cut back on empty calories:

Choose foods and drinks with little or no added sugars or solid fats.
For example, drink water instead of sugary drinks. There

are about 10 packets of sugar in a 12-ounce can of soda, while water has no added sugars.

Select lean cuts of meats or poultry and fat-free or low-fat milk and cheese. Fatty meats, poultry skin, and whole milk or regular cheese have more solid fats.

Select products that contain added sugars and solid fats *less often*.

For example, eat sugary desserts only once in a while. Most days, select fruit for dessert instead of a sugary option.

Make major sources of solid fats – such as cakes, cookies, ice cream, pizza, regular cheese, sausages, and hot dogs – occasional choices, not every day foods.

When you have foods and drinks with added sugars and solid fats, choose a small portion.

For example, instead of eating three scoops of ice cream, order one scoop.

Concerned about eating fewer empty calories? Here are some common "stumbling blocks" and ideas to help you overcome these barriers:

"Empty calories aren't listed on food labels. How do I know how many are in my foods and beverages?": While empty calories are not listed on the food label, you can use the label to see if there are solid fats and added sugars in the food.

"I don't understand if I should focus on total calories or empty calories": Foods that are high in empty calories tend to be high in total calories too. It is the total amount of calories consumed each day that can affect weight. If you currently eat too many empty calories, eating

"When I get the cravings for something sweet, I just can't help myself!": Replace foods high in empty calories with better choices. For example, try a yogurt parfait with low-fat or fat-free yogurt and sliced fruit or frozen grapes for a sweet treat. You can still get the sweet you want without the excess calories.

8. Focus on Foods You Need

Building a healthier plate can help you meet your nutrient needs and maintain your weight. Foods like vegetables, fruits, whole grains, low-fat dairy products, and lean protein foods contain the nutrients you need without too many calories.

When making food choices, use your Daily Food Plan (https://www.choosemyplate.gov/MyPlate-Daily-Checklist). Focus on the 5 food groups. Most of what you eat and drink each day should fit within one or more of the 5 food groups. To move to a healthier weight, you need to make **smart choices** from every food group. Smart choices are the foods with low amounts of solid fats or added sugars: such as, fat-free (skim) milk instead of whole milk, unsweetened applesauce instead of sweetened applesauce, and 95% lean ground beef instead of regular (75% lean) ground beef.

Also think about how the food was prepared. For example, choose skinless baked chicken instead of fried chicken and choose fresh fruit instead of a fruit pastry. You can learn more about making smart choices within the food groups by going to the Food Groups (https://www.choosemyplate.gov/MyPlate) section. Focusing on the foods you need can help you eat a healthy diet and manage weight.

Does it matter how much carbohydrate, protein, and fat you eat? Carbohydrate, protein, and fat are components of foods and drinks that provide calories. "Calories" matter when it comes to body weight, not the calorie source. You should not select a diet that avoids or severely limits carbohydrates, protein, or fat. Similarly, you should not select a diet that avoids any of the 5 food groups. There are choices within each food group that provide the nutrients you need, without too many calories.

Get Started focusing on the foods you need:

Start with breakfast. Eat a breakfast that helps you meet your food group needs. People who skip breakfast often weigh more. Eating a nutrient-dense breakfast may help you lose weight and keep it off.

Have healthy snacks available at home and bring healthy snacks to eat when on-the-go, such as carrot and celery sticks with peanut butter or whole grain crackers and low-fat cheese.

When preparing meals, include vegetables, fruits, whole grains, fat-free or low-fat dairy products, and lean protein foods. These foods provide nutrients with fewer calories.

To feel satisfied with fewer calories, replace high-calorie foods with lower calorie foods. You can eat larger portions of these foods for fewer calories. For example, follow the advice to *"make half your plate fruits and vegetables."*

Concerned about focusing on the foods you need? Here are some common "stumbling blocks" and ideas to help you overcome these barriers:

"I don't like many vegetables." or "I don't eat fruit": Explore the wide range of different vegetables that are available and choose some you're willing to try. If you're not fond of cooked vegetables, experiment with salads and raw vegetables. Or, try mixed dishes that include vegetables, like stir-fries, chili con carne, vegetable soups, or pasta with marinara sauce. When eating out, choose a vegetable (other than french fries) as a side dish. For fruits, try adding fruit to salads, making fruit smoothies, or snacking on dried fruit.

"I don't/can't drink milk": You don't need to drink milk, but you do need the nutrients it provides. You can get these nutrients from yogurt, from fortified soymilk (soy beverage), or from low-fat cheese. Milk or other foods from the Dairy Group can also be incorporated into lots of foods and drinks including lattes, puddings, and soups. Try some new ways to include milk or other foods from the Dairy Group in your meals and snacks.

"My family members don't like these foods. I'm worried about spending the time and money preparing them if they don't get eaten": Be patient when introducing new foods to your family. It may take more than a few tries before the new food is accepted. Also, be a good role model. If you like the food and you show that you like it, your family is more likely to like it too. Also, encourage family members to pick out a new food to try. If you have leftovers, portion them out and freeze them for another day.

"Fruits and vegetables are too expensive": It is possible to fit vegetables and fruits into any budget. Buy fresh fruits and vegetables that are in season; they are easy to get, have more flavor, and are usually less expensive. You can also try canned or frozen. For canned items, choose fruit canned in 100% fruit juice and vegetables with "low sodium" or "no salt added" on the label. And don't forget to check the local newspaper, online, and at the store for sales, coupons, and specials that will cut food costs.

9. When Eating Out, Make Better Choices

How often do you eat out? Once a day? Once a week? Rarely? Almost every meal? People who eat out more often, particularly at fast food restaurants, are more likely to be overweight or obese. However, you can still manage your body weight when eating out by making better choices.

To eat out without blowing your calorie budget, there are three things to think about:

WHAT you are eating and drinking,

HOW MUCH you are eating and drinking, and

HOW your meal is prepared.

Get Started making better choices when eating out:

What are you eating and drinking?

Check posted calorie amounts, and choose lower calorie menu options. Many restaurants post calories on menus, in pamphlets, or on their websites. Compare food and beverage options and think about how they fit within your daily calorie limit (https://www.choosemyplate.gov/MyPlate-Daily-Checklist). For example, if your daily calorie limit is 1600 calories, think twice before ordering a meal with 1300 calories. Also, don't forget about the calories from drinks, dressings, dips, appetizers, and desserts. They all count!

Choose dishes that include vegetables, fruits, whole grains, low-fat dairy products, and lean protein foods. Focusing on smart food choices from each of the 5 food groups can help you stay on track at restaurants.

Think about what you drink. Ask for water or order fat-free or low-fat milk, unsweetened tea, or other drinks without added sugars. If you choose to drink alcoholic beverages, select options with fewer calories. For example, a frozen Pinacolada or margarita can have over 400 calories! Watch out for desserts. Some restaurants are serving small portions of desserts, which can help decrease calorie intake. However, as a good rule, eat dessert less often.

How much are you eating and drinking?

Avoid oversized portions. A major challenge for many people when they eat out is being served large portions. Most people eat and drink more when served larger portions. To overcome this challenge, choose a smaller size option, share your meal, or take home half of your meal. For example, hamburgers can range from as few as 250 calories to 800 calories or more. Choose a smaller option with fewer calories.

To help you eat less when eating out, order from the menu instead of heading for the all-you-can-eat buffet. Many people overeat at buffets. Getting a plate of food, instead of unlimited access to food, may help you eat less. Don't forget that you don't have to clean your plate!

How is your meal prepared?

Order steamed, grilled, or broiled dishes instead of those that are fried or sauteéd. Avoid choosing foods with the following words: creamy, breaded, battered, or buttered. These words indicate that the food is higher in calories.

Ask for dressings, sauces, and syrups "on the side" so you can add only as much as you want. These sides are often high in calories – so don't eat much of them.

Concerned about **making better choices when eating out**? Here are some common "stumbling blocks" and ideas to help you overcome these barriers:

"I feel that I have to eat everything on my plate since it is there in front of me or else I feel like I'm wasting food": To control how much you eat, ask for a take home box with your order, and box half of the food up as soon as it arrives. This way you know that you will have saved on calories and also have a delicious lunch for the following day.

"I like to have a cocktail with dinner": Moderate alcohol consumption can be a part of a healthy diet. Limit alcohol to no more than 1 drink per day for women and 2 drinks per day for men. Don't forget that some drinks provide a lot of calories. Many alcoholic beverages range from 100 to 400 calories each.

"I have heard that salads can be worse for you than a

big meal!": Salads can be high in calories if they have toppings like fried chicken, loads of cheese, and creamy dressing. To start a meal, choose a salad that is all vegetables, and ask for dressing on the side. For a main dish salad, choose one with topped with grilled or baked chicken, seafood, or lean beef.

"It's a tradition now to get dessert after our meals when we eat out.": Ask your friends or family to support your efforts to eat less by understanding that you won't be ordering dessert. While they eat dessert, have a cup of tea or coffee. Have one bite of someone's dessert if they offer to share. If fruit is available as a dessert option, order it without the whipped topping or sauce.

10. Cook More Often at Home

Over the last few decades, Americans have been eating out more and cooking at home less often. When you cook at home, you can often make better choices about what and how much you eat and drink than you do when eating out. Cooking can also be a fun activity and a way for you to spend time with family and friends.

When cooking remember to Focus on Foods You Need, Eat Fewer Empty Calories, and Decrease Portion Sizes. Many recipes include calorie content per serving. Compare calorie content and choose meals that fit within your daily calorie needs. If cooking for a family, you may each have different calorie needs. You can still cook the same nutritious foods, but vary the portion sizes. For example, an active adolescent male can still eat the same foods as his five-year-old sister, he will just eat more.

Get started cooking more often at home:

If you don't usually cook, start gradually. Make it a goal to cook once a week and work up to cooking more often.

A healthy meal starts with more vegetables and fruits and smaller portions of protein and grains. Think about how you can adjust the portions on your plate to get more of what you need without too many calories. And don't forget dairy – make it the beverage with your meal or add fat-free or low-fat dairy products to your plate. You don't have to eat from every food group at each meal, but thinking about the food groups can help you build a healthy meal. Planning ahead can help you make better food choices. Keep healthy staples on hand, such as dried fruit, whole wheat pasta, "no-salt-added" canned vegetables, and frozen seafood.

Look for ways to make your favorite recipes healthier. For example, use the low-fat or reduced-fat version of dairy products like cheese and milk or replace sour-cream with low-fat or fat-free yogurt. Also use spices and herbs to add more flavor instead of adding salt or fat.

To help manage how much you eat, start by putting a small portion of food on your plate, and only eat seconds if still hungry.

Concerned **about cooking more often at home?** Here are some common "stumbling blocks" and ideas to help you overcome these barriers:

"I'm tired of being the only one that cooks": Make cooking a family event. Get your children involved with the prep work. This will help to teach them about healthy eating, and it also serves as a way for you to spend time with your children. Have an occasional potluck. Invite friends over and have everyone bring their favorite healthy dish.

"I don't have time to cook a big meal every night; it is easier to just order out": Cooking does take time, but there are several things that you can do to make it easier to cook at home. Try prepping dishes the night before, or the morning of; prepping the salad or the side dish can help save time after work. Also try cooking a big meal on Sunday and then eating it as leftovers and freezing extras. Buying frozen or canned fruits and vegetables can also save prep time.

"My family prefers to eat out; when I cook at home, they complain": Changing a family pattern is difficult at first. Start by eating one more meal at home each week than you normally do. You may save calories and money! To mix things up, try a new recipe.

11. Increase Physical Activity

Physical activity is an important part of managing body weight.

Being physically active can help you achieve a healthy weight and prevent excess weight gain. However, physical activity is also important to all other aspects of your health. Benefits include sleeping better at night, decreasing your chances of becoming depressed, and helping you look good. When you are not physically active, you are more likely to have health problems, including heart disease, type 2 diabetes, and high blood cholesterol.

The amount of physical activity needed to manage body weight depends on calorie intake and varies a lot from person to person. Some adults will need to do more physical activity than others to manage body weight.

How much physical activity do you need to help manage body weight?

To start, adults should do the equivalent of 150 minutes (2 hours and 30 minutes) of moderate-intensity aerobic activity each week.

If necessary, adults should increase their weekly minutes of aerobic physical activity gradually over time (while eating fewer calories) to meet weight loss goals.

Some adults who need to lose weight may need to do more than the equivalent of 300 minutes (5 hours) per week of moderate-intensity activity to meet weight loss goals.

This may sound like a lot. However, your weight is a balance of the number of calories you eat and drink and the physical activity you do. Weight loss can be achieved by eating and drinking fewer calories OR by burning more calories in physical activity. The people with the greatest long-term success are doing BOTH – eating less and being more active. For example, walking 30 minutes each day and drinking one less soda each day are two small steps you can take that can have a big impact on your weight over time.

Get started increasing physical activity:

Pick activities you like and that fit into your life.

Be active with family and friends. Having a support network can help you stay active.

Keep track of your physical activity and gradually increase how much you do over time. Use the SuperTracker (https://www.supertracker.usda.gov/), a journal, or mark your activity on a calendar.

Concerned about increasing physical activity? Here are some common "stumbling blocks" and ideas to help you overcome these barriers:

"I dislike physical activity. Running just isn't my idea of fun": Pick activities that you like and start by doing what you can, at least 10 minutes at a time. Every bit adds up, and the health benefits increase as you spend more time being active. If one activity, like running, doesn't appeal to you, find something that does. There are lots of activities, such as: swimming, biking, walking, playing tennis, basketball, hiking, rollerblading, etc. The point is to get out there and move! Doing something is better than doing nothing.

"I don't have the energy to be active": Daily activities like walking, gardening, and climbing up the stairs all count. Start with what you can do, even if that's just 10 minutes. You may even find yourself more energized after being active!

"I don't know the first thing about being active": Physical activity simply means movement of the body that uses energy. You can choose moderate or vigorous intensity activities, or a mix of both, each week. Moderate physical activities include: walking briskly, bicycling, dancing, and golf. Vigorous physical activities include: running, jogging, swimming, basketball, and aerobics.

"How do I know when I have gotten enough exercise for the day?": For substantial health benefits, the Physical Activity Guidelines recommend that adults get at least 150 minutes (2 hours and 30 minutes) a week of moderate-intensity activity or 75 minutes (1 hour and 15 minutes) a week of vigorous-intensity aerobic physical activity, or an equivalent combination of moderate- and vigorous-intensity aerobic activity. Aerobic activity should be performed in episodes of at least 10 minutes, and preferably, it should be spread throughout the week.

12. Decrease Television and Computer Time

To help manage your body weight, reduce the amount of time you spend being sedentary. This includes time spent in front of a screen - including watching television, playing video games, and using the computer.

People who spend more time being sedentary, particularly watching television, are more likely to be overweight or obese.

Most people can't change how much time they spend on the computer for work or school, but you can decrease your screen time during other times of the day and on the weekend.

Get started decreasing television and computer time:

Track how much time you spend in front of a screen. Log the number of hours you spend in a week (outside of work or school) watching television, playing video games, or using the computer.

Develop a screen time budget. Set a goal to reduce screen time. Plan to watch shows you'd like to see. Write down a few options of things you could do instead of watching television, like taking a walk around the block, gardening, or playing with your dog.

Use the time you watch television to be physically active in front of the television. Walk in place (or on a treadmill) while watching your favorite shows, or do jumping jacks during commercials.

Limit eating while watching television. Many people overeat when watching television because they aren't thinking about what they are eating - they stop eating when the bowl or bag is empty, instead of when they have had enough! If you choose to eat while watching television, portion out a small amount.

Concerned about decreasing Television and Computer time? Here are some common "stumbling blocks" and ideas to help you overcome these barriers:

"I'm exhausted after work and just want to sit on the sofa!": It can be difficult to break your routine. Start by making small changes. For example, do you watch three hours of television most nights? Try cutting out just one program, and use the time to take a walk or play with the kids. Find activities that you enjoy and will look forward to – anything that gets you moving. Being active with family or friends can help you create a healthy new routine.

"I like to play video games that have an active component, like yoga or tennis. Do those count as screen time?": Some active video games count as physical activity. Limit the amount of time you spend **inactive** in front of the television, including video games. Playing an active video game can be a fun way to get physical activity. The activity should make your heart beat faster and your breathing rate pick up for it to count as physical activity.

"I've logged my screen time, but I can't figure out how much TV time I should set as my goal. Are there recommendations that I can follow?": Try limiting your total screen time to 2 hours a day (outside of work or school). Start by picking your favorite shows that you want to watch. Find other activities, such as walking, or find a new hobby that you enjoy doing in place of watching television.

13. How to Build a Healthy Meal

A healthy meal starts with more vegetables and fruits and smaller portions of protein and grains. Think about how you can adjust the portions on your plate to get more of what you need without too many calories. And don't forget dairy—make it the beverage with your meal or add fat-free or low-fat dairy products to your plate.

Make half your plate veggies and fruits Vegetables and fruits are full of nutrients and may help to promote good health. Choose red, orange, and dark-green vegetables such as tomatoes, sweet potatoes, and broccoli.

Add lean protein

Choose protein foods, such as lean beef and pork, or chicken, turkey, beans, or tofu. Twice a week, make seafood the protein on your plate.

Include whole grains

Aim to make at least half your grains whole grains. Look for the words "100% whole grain" or "100% whole wheat" on the food label. Whole grains provide more nutrients, like fiber, than refined grains.

Don't forget the dairy

Pair your meal with a cup of fat-free or low-fat milk. They

provide the same amount of calcium and other essential nutrients as whole milk, but less fat and calories. Don't drink milk? Try soymilk (soy beverage) as your beverage or include

Avoid extra fat

Using heavy gravies or sauces will add fat and calories to otherwise healthy choices. For example, steamed broccoli is great, but avoid topping it with cheese sauce. Try other options, like a sprinkling of low-fat parmesan cheese or a squeeze of lemon.

Take your time

Savor your food. Eat slowly, enjoy the taste and textures, and pay attention to how you feel. Be mindful. Eating very quickly may cause you to eat too much.

Use a smaller plate

Use a smaller plate at meals to help with portion control. That way you can finish your entire plate and feel satisfied without overeating.

Take control of your food

Eat at home more often so you know exactly what you are eating. If you eat out, check and compare the nutrition information. Choose healthier options such as baked instead of fried.

Try new foods

Keep it interesting by picking out new foods you've never tried before, like mango, lentils, or kale. You may find a new favorite! Trade fun and tasty recipes with friends or find them online.

Satisfy your sweet tooth in a healthy way

Indulge in a naturally sweet dessert dish—fruit! Serve a fresh fruit cocktail or a fruit parfait made with yogurt. For a hot dessert, bake apples and top with cinnamon.

14. How to Keep Eating Healthy Food While on a Budget

There are many ways to save money on the foods that you eat. The three main steps are planning before you shop, purchasing the items at the best price, and preparing meals that stretch your food dollars.

Plan, plan, plan!

Before you head to the grocery store, plan your meals for the week. Include meals like stews, casseroles, or sitr-fries, which "stretch" expensive items into more portions. Check to see what foods you already have and make a list for what you need to buy.

Get the best price

Check the local newspaper, online, and at the store for sales and coupons. Ask about a loyalty card for extra savings at stores where you shop. Look for specials or sales on meat and seafood—often the most expensive items on your list.

Compare and contrast

Locate the "Unit Price" on the shelf directly below the product. Use it to compare different brands and different sizes of the same brand to determine which is more economical.

Buy in bulk

It is almost always cheaper to buy foods in bulk. Smart choices are family packs of chicken, steak, or fish and larger bags of potatoes and frozen vegetables. Before you shop, remember to check if you have enough freezer space.

Buy in season

Buying fruits and vegetables in season can lower the cost and add to the freshness! If you are not going to use them all right away, buy some that still need time to ripen.

Convenience costs... go back to the basics

Convenience foods like frozen dinners, pre-cut vegetables, and instant rice, oatmeal, or grits will cost you more than if you were to make them from scratch yourself. Take the time to prepare your own—and save!

Easy on your wallet

Certain foods are typically low-cost options all year round. Try beans for a less expensive protein food. For vegetables, buy carrots, greens, or potatoes. As for fruits, apples and bananas are good choices.

Cook once...eat all week!

Prepare a large batch of favorite recipes on your day off (double or triple the recipe). Freeze in individual containers. Use them throughout the week and you won't have to spend money on take-out meals.

Get your creative juices flowing

Spice up your leftovers—use them in new ways. For example, try leftover chicken in a stir-fry or over a garden salad, or to make chicken chili. Remember,

Eating out

Restaurants can be expensive. Save money by getting the early bird special, going out for lunch instead of dinner, or looking for "2 for 1" deals. Stick to water instead of ordering other beverages, which add to the bill.

15. The Only Way To Start a Diet That Really Works

Losing weight takes more than desire. It takes commitment and a well-thought-out plan. Here's a step-by-step guide to getting started.

Step 1: Make a commitment.

Making the decision to lose weight, change your lifestyle, and become healthier is a big step to take. Start simply by making a commitment to yourself. Many people find it helpful to sign a written contract committing to the process. This contract may include things like the amount of weight you want to lose, the date you'd like to lose the weight by, the dietary changes you'll make to establish healthy eating habits, and a plan for getting regular physical activity.

Writing down the reasons why you want to lose weight can also help. It might be because you have a family history of heart disease, or because you want to see your kids get married, or simply because you want to feel better in your clothes. Post these reasons where they serve as a daily reminder of why you want to make this change.

Step 2: Take stock of where you are.

Consider talking to your health care provider. He or she can evaluate your height, weight, and explore other weight-related risk factors you may have. Ask for a follow-up appointment to monitor changes in your weight or any related health conditions.

Keep a "food diary" for a few days, in which you write down everything you eat. By doing this, you become more aware of what you are eating and when you are eating. This awareness can help you avoid mindless eating.

Next, examine your current lifestyle. Identify things that might pose challenges to your weight loss efforts. For example, does your work or travel schedule make it difficult to get enough physical activity? Do you find yourself eating sugary foods because that's what you buy for your kids? Do your coworkers frequently bring high-calorie items, such as donats, to the workplace to share with everyone? Think through things you can do to help overcome these challenges.

Finally, think about aspects of your lifestyle that can help you lose weight. For example, is there an area near your workplace where you and some coworkers can take a walk at lunchtime? Is there a place in your community, such as a YMCA, with exercise facilities for you and child care for your kids?

Step 3: Set realistic goals.

Set some short-term goals and reward your efforts along the way. If your long-term goal is to lose 40 pounds and to control your high blood pressure, some short-term eating and physical activity goals might be to start eating breakfast, taking a 15 minute walk in the evenings, or having a salad or vegetable with supper.

Focus on two or three goals at a time. Great, effective goals are —

Specific

Realistic

Forgiving (less than perfect)

For example, "Exercise More" is not a specific goal. But if you say, "I will walk 15 minutes, 3 days a week for the first week," you are setting a specific and realistic goal for the first week.

Remember, small changes every day can lead to big results in the long run. Also remember that realistic goals are achievable goals. By achieving your short-term goals day-by-day, you'll feel good about your progress and be motivated to continue. Setting unrealistic goals, such as losing 20 pounds in 2 weeks, can leave you feeling defeated and frustrated.

Being realistic also means expecting occasional setbacks. Setbacks happen when you get away from your plan for whatever reason – maybe the holidays, longer work hours, or another life change. When setbacks happen, get back on track as quickly as possible. Also take some time to think about what you would do differently if a similar situation happens, to prevent setbacks.

Keep in mind everyone is different – what works for

someone else might not be right for you. Just because your neighbor lost weight by taking up running, doesn't mean running is the best option for you. Try a variety of activities – walking, swimming, tennis, or group exercise classes to see what you enjoy most and can fit into your life. These activities will be easier to stick with over the long term.

Step 4: Identify resources for information and support.

Find family members or friends who will support your weight loss efforts. Making lifestyle changes can feel easier when you have others you can talk to and rely on for support. You might have coworkers or neighbors with similar goals, and together you can share healthful recipes and plan group exercise.

Joining a weight loss group or visiting a health care professional such as a registered dietitian, can help.

Step 5: Continually "check in" with yourself to monitor your progress.

Revisit the goals you set for yourself (in Step 3) and evaluate your progress regularly. If you set a goal to walk each morning but are having trouble fitting it in before work, see if you can shift your work hours or if you can get your walk in at lunchtime or after work. Evaluate which parts of your plan are working well and which ones need tweaking. Then rewrite your goals and plan accordingly.

If you are consistently achieving a particular goal, add a new goal to help you continue on your pathway to success.

Reward yourself for your successes! Recognize when you're meeting your goals and be proud of your progress. Use non-food rewards, such as a bouquet of freshly picked flowers, a sports outing with friends, or a relaxing bath. Rewards help keep you motivated on the path to better health.

16. Are You Following These Essential Weight Loss Ideas?

Making food choices for a healthy lifestyle can be as simple as using these 10 ideas. Use the ideas in this list to balance your calories, to choose foods to eat more often, and to cut back on foods to eat less often.

1. switch to fat-free or low-fat (1%) milk - They have the same amount of calcium and other essential nutrients as whole milk, but fewer calories and less saturated fat.

2. make half your grains whole grains - To eat more whole grains, substitute a whole-grain product for a refined product—such as eating whole wheat bread instead of white bread or brown rice instead of white rice.

3. foods to eat less often - Cut back on foods high in solid fats, added sugars, and salt. They include cakes, cookies, ice cream, candies, sweetened drinks, pizza, and fatty meats like ribs, sausages, bacon, and hot dogs. Use these foods as occasional treats, not everyday foods.

4. compare sodium in foods - Use the Nutrition Facts label to choose lower sodium versions of foods like soup, bread, and frozen meals. Select canned foods labeled "low sodium," "reduced sodium," or "no salt added."

5. drink water instead of sugary drinks - Cut calories by drinking water or unsweetened beverages. Soda, energy

drinks, and sports drinks are a major source of added sugar, and calories, in American diets.

6. make half your plate fruits and vegetables - Choose red, orange, and dark-green vegetables like tomatoes, sweet potatoes, and broccoli, along with other vegetables for your meals. Add fruit to meals as part of main or side dishes or as dessert.

7. balance calories - Find out how many calories YOU need for a day as a first step in managing your weight. Being physically active also helps you balance calories.

8. enjoy your food, but eat less - Take the time to fully enjoy your food as you eat it. Eating too fast or when your attention is elsewhere may lead to eating too many calories. Pay attention to hunger and fullness cues before, during, and after meals. Use them to recognize when to eat and when you've had enough.

9. avoid oversized portions - Use a smaller plate, bowl, and glass. Portion out foods before you eat. When eating out, choose a smaller size option, share a dish, or take home part of your meal.

10. foods to eat more often - Eat more vegetables, fruits, whole grains, and fat-free or 1% milk and dairy products. These foods have the nutrients you need for health—including potassium, calcium, vitamin D, and fiber. Make them the basis for meals and snacks.

17. How To Break a Weight Loss Plateau Without Starving Yourself

As anyone who has ever lost a lot of weight will tell you, the first 5 pounds come off easily and the last 5 are the toughest! You're still doing all the right things - eating less and moving more - but all of a sudden it stops working. The scale won't budge. No matter where you are in the process, hitting a stubborn weight loss plateau is frustrating. But don't let it erode your resolve. Here are 5 quick tips to break through the plateau:

1. Adjust your caloric intake, you may be eating too few or too many.

2. Start measuring portions - they tend to get larger when we get used to eyeballing them.

3. Drink more water, eat less salt, refined sugar and refined grains.

4. Add new exercises into your routine - up the intensity of your workout.

5. Add strength training to your routine - it will boost your metabolism.

And now here are some general weight loss tips of interest from this week's crop:

Try to avoid fad diets. Many of these are not tailored to fit everybody's different nutritional and health-related needs, so doing some of these without consulting a physician can be dangerous. many leave out important daily nutrients that your body needs. Stick to things like lean meats, watching your fats, cholesterol and sugars, and eating healthy produce with a lot of water.

Put a lot of fiber in your diet. Foods with a lot of fiber in them such as nuts and whole-grains are great. Because the fiber takes a long time to break down in the body, you feel full for longer than with other foods. This way you won't have cravings for junk food as often.

Milk is the best form of liquid protein you can give you body. Packed full of protein, vitamin D and other important nutrients, milk is a natural, affordable drink, that everyone should take advantage of. Instead of using protein shakes to bulk up, consider drinking two or three glasses of milk every day, instead.

As you grocery shop, make sure your children are involved in the process. Let them choose which fruits and vegetables they want to eat. Doing this can also entice children to try out new foods, especially those with bright colors.

A great nutrition tip is to start incorporating flax seed into your diet. Flax seed is an amazing source of essential fatty acids and it's very easy to add to food. You can sprinkle a bit of flax seed in your protein shake, or you can put a little bit in your salad.

If you are a vegetarian, make sure your nutrition choices are well-rounded. While many omnivores miss essential vitamins in their diet, it's easier to recover lost minerals. That said, it's easy to keep on top of a vegetarian diet. If you find yourself hitting roadblocks, consider seeing a nutritionist.

18. Do You Make This Common Weight Loss Mistake?

The single most critical mistake dieters do is setting unrealistic goals. In order to lose weight in a healthy, sustainable way you should aim to subtract no more than 500 to 1000 calories daily, this translates into losing about 1 to 2 pounds a week respectively (about 0.5kg to 1kg).

Keep in mind that setting realistic goals and tracking your progress are key to your success. Research has shown that those who keep track of their behaviors are more likely to take off weight. As a matter of fact, setting unrealistic diet goals is the main reason most diets fail. You want to develop lifestyle habits that will help you maintain your weight in a healthy range. A short-term "diet" that you "go on" and then "go off" is not the answer to long-term weight management.

Now here are some more tips to help you with your weight loss efforts:

1. To make a delicious low fat mayonnaise simply combine one teaspoon Dijon mustard or one teaspoon Satay sauce with low fat yogurt.

2. Avoid skipping meals. Eating increases your metabolism, thus skipping meals can 'trick' your body into slowing down its metabolism in an attempt to conserve calories

during a period it perceives as a situation where limited fuel is available.

3. Stuffing vegetables such as capsicum and zucchini with tasty fillings of mince chicken, meat or tuna are easy to do and very healthy and low fat.

4. Pita bread roll ups or wraps with salad fillings, are great for picnics, school lunches or to take to work.

5. Exercise, exercise, exercise! Exercise increases your metabolism and burning off excess fat. When is the best time to exercise? Our metabolism slows down about 8 hours after we wake up, so 30 minutes of exercise in the evening, before dinner will increase your metabolism for about two to three more hours just when it was starting to slow down. This produces a significant increase in fat burned off, even after the exercise is over.

6. Adding alfalfa or Mung beans to your salad brings in extra iron.

7. Good cooking and healthy eating begins with learning about nutrition and how to prepare healthy recipes.

8. Plan the week's family menus in advance and just purchase those ingredients at a once weekly shopping trip.

9. Be positive! The more you feel good about yourself the easier and faster it is to lose weight.

10. Learn how to make over family favorite recipes by cutting out fats, salt and sugar. Substitute non fat yogurt for

cream, stir fry minus oil and use herbs and spices instead of salt for flavor.

11. Please consult your doctor before beginning an exercise or weight loss program.

12. Eat slowly and chew each bite completely to decrease your appetite.

13. Eat three small meals and two snacks daily instead of two or three huge meals.

14. It's a myth that you need oil to stir fry! Use chicken stock instead and cut down on hidden fat.

15. There is more fat in a plate of toasted muesli than a plate of bacon and eggs! Purchase non-toasted muesli instead.

16. Avoid removing the skins of fruits and vegetables - most of the nutrients are concentrated just under the skin.

17. Hot water with a squeeze of lemon before breakfast get the metabolism going for the day, helps prevent constipation and is excellent for the skin.

18. The best source of vegetable protein is from soya beans or tofu. All legumes provide some protein, so include lentils, Lima beans etc into casseroles and soups.

19. Find a weight loss "buddy," club, or support group. This will help you stay with your weight loss program.

20. Though difficult, try not eating 3 hours or more before

bed time.

21. Cut up a whole watermelon and leave it in the fridge to snack on over a few days. it is sweet, juicy, yummy and filling. it really has helped me because when I go to the fridge looking for something when i see the watermelon it stops me having something more calorie laden. having it handy so that it is just as easy to eat as a biscuit or whatever makes the world of difference. eating at night time is my downfall too. I can't just not eat at night so I allow for it in my daily eating. I have those 97% fat free rice crackers and/or fruit or air popped popcorn. for me I just can't not eat at night time. I find I don't sleep very well if I go from dinner time to breakfast without anything. Although we do eat dinner very early (around 6:00) because we like to eat with the kids. I think it is best to know your weaknesses and try to work around them. also, I don't think it can be said too many times - drinking water makes all the difference.

22. Make pasta your fast food choice - you can prepare a pasta meal and salad in 10-12 minutes.

23. Chili helps to speed up metabolism - even the milder varieties.

24. Omelets can be made just using egg whites! A dramatic reduction in fat.

25. Limit salt in cooking. Other names for salt include baking soda, baking powder, MSG and soya sauce.

26. For low fat gravy, drop ice cubes into the baking tray. Fat will stick to the ice cubes and can then be removed.

27. Chew sugarless gum. It speeds up the digestive system, burning more calories, and sometimes kills a craving.

28. Drinking hot water as appose to cold water can increase the speed of your metabolism and burn more calories.

29. Make casseroles the day before use. Refrigerate and skim fat from the top before re-heating.

30. Always eat before you go food shopping and always prepare a shopping list. Only purchase food which relates to your weekly menu plan and don't be tempted to buy goodies.

19. How To Keep The Pounds Off Without Gaining Them Back

If you've recently lost excess weight, congratulations! It's an accomplishment that will likely benefit your health now and in the future. Now that you've lost weight, let's talk about some ways to maintain that success.

When you lose weight, especially a significant amount, it's cause for celebration. But if those pounds gradually reappear, you've achieved only a hollow victory.

The following tips are some of the common characteristics among people who have successfully lost weight and maintained that loss over time.

Watch Your Diet

Follow a healthy and realistic eating pattern. You have embarked on a healthier lifestyle, now the challenge is maintaining the positive eating habits you've developed along the way. In studies of people who have lost weight and kept it off for at least a year, most continued to eat a diet lower in calories as compared to their pre-weight loss diet.

Keep your eating patterns consistent. Follow a healthy eating pattern regardless of changes in your routine. Plan ahead for weekends, vacations, and special occasions. By making a plan, it is more likely you'll have healthy foods on hand for when your routine changes.

Eat breakfast every day. Eating breakfast is a common trait among people who have lost weight and kept it off. Eating a healthful breakfast may help you avoid getting "over-hungry" and then overeating later in the day.

Be Active

Get daily physical activity. People who have lost weight and kept it off typically engage in 20—60 minutes of moderate intensity physical activity most days of the week while not exceeding calorie needs. This doesn't necessarily mean 60 minutes at one time. It might mean 20 minutes of physical activity three times a day. For example, a brisk walk in the morning, at lunch time, and in the evening. Some people may need to talk to their healthcare provider before participating in this level of physical activity.

Stay on Course

Monitor your diet and activity. Keeping a food and physical activity journal can help you track your progress and spot trends. For example, you might notice that your weight creeps up during periods when you have a lot of business travel or when you have to work overtime. Recognizing this tendency can be a signal to try different behaviors, such as packing your own healthful food for the plane and making time to use your hotel's exercise facility when you are traveling. Or if working overtime, maybe you can use your breaks for quick walks around the building.

Monitor your weight. Check your weight regularly. When managing your weight loss, it's a good idea to keep track of your weight so you can plan accordingly and adjust your diet and exercise plan as necessary. If you have gained a few pounds, get back on track quickly.

Get support from family, friends, and others. People who have successfully lost weight and kept it off often rely on support from others to help them stay on course and get over any "bumps." Sometimes having a friend or partner who is also losing weight or maintaining a weight loss can help you stay motivated.

20. Keep Your Weight Down With These Mouth Watering Snacks

Snacking is good when you feel hungry between meals. Choosing healthy snacks will help you and your family stay at a healthy weight.

Each of these snacks is in the 200 calorie range so you can snack guilt free while trimming down. Even mix and match the snacks to create tasty, new combinations!

1. 30 pistachios.

2. 2 Hard boiled eggs.

3. 1/2 small bagel + 1oz smoked salmon + 1 tbsp cream cheese

4. cup steamed edamame beans.

5. 1 medium apple sliced + 2 tsp peanut butter

6. 1 cup 1% milk + 2 tbsp chocolate syrup.

7. 3 cups cheddar popcorn.

8. 1/2 cup low fat yogurt + 2 tsp honey + 1 tsp cocoa powder + 1/2 cup raspberries.

9. 1/2 apple + 1 slice cheddar cheese.

10. 3 tbsp chocolate chips + 8 pistachios.

11. 1 cup red bell pepper slices + 1/2 cup refried beans + 2 tbsp guacamole.

12. 25 almonds.

13. 1 avocado.

14. 1 slice banana nut bread

15. 1/2 English muffin + 2 tbsp cream cheese.

16. 1/2 cup frozen yogurt.

17. 1/2 English muffin + slice of tomato + slice of mozzarella.

18. 6 oz Greek yogurt + 1 cup strawberries.

19. 1 medium apple +1 stick cheese.

20. 10 carrot sticks + 2 tbsp dip.

21. 8 tortilla chips + 1/2 cup salsa.

22. 4 oz 1% cottage cheese + 3/4 cup fresh fruit.

23. 5 whole wheat crackers + 1 oz cheese.

24. 1/4 cup hummus + 1 cup raw veggies.

25. 1 large bunch of red grapes (about 50).

26. 20 Kalamata olives.

Here Is Another List of Healthy Snacks, This One In The Range of 100 Calories or Less

Fruits

1 small banana

1 medium apple

¼ cup raisins

1 cup whole strawberries

½ cup canned fruit cocktail in juice (not syrup)

½ cup orange juice

Vegetables

1 cup cherry or grape tomatoes

2 cups raw mixed veggies with 2 tablespoons fat-free dressing

12 baby carrots

18 small celery sticks

1 cup raw cauliflower

1 cup low-sodium vegetable juice

Breads, Cereals, Rice, and Pasta

½ cup oat circles cereal

2 graham cracker squares

3 cups air-popped popcorn

½ whole-wheat English muffin with jelly

4 whole-wheat crackers, unsalted

2 brown rice and multi-grain rice cakes

Fat-free or Low-fat Milk, Cheese, and Yogurt

6 ounces cup fat-free plain yogurt

½ cup low-fat cottage cheese

1 cup fat-free milk

½ cup fat-free pudding

½ cup fat-free frozen yogurt

1 ounce low-fat cheddar cheese

Other Snacks

1 large hardboiled egg

8 baked tortilla chips with salsa

10 almonds

21. Don't Be Fooled By These 11 Weight Loss Myths

"Lose 30 pounds in 30 days!"

"Eat as much as you want and still lose weight!"

"Try the thigh buster and lose inches fast!"

Have you heard these claims before? A large number of diets and tools are available, but their quality may vary. It can be hard to know what to believe.

This fact sheet may help. Here, we discuss myths and provide facts and tips about weight loss, nutrition, and physical activity. This information may help you make healthy changes in your daily habits.

Weight-loss and Diet Myths

Myth: Fad diets will help me lose weight and keep it off.

Healthy habits may help you lose weight.

 Make healthy food choices. Half of your plate should be fruits and veggies.

Eat small portions. Use a smaller plate, weigh portions on a scale, or check the Nutrition Facts label for details about serving sizes (see below).

 Build exercise into your daily life. Garden, go for family walks, play a pickup game of sports, start a dance club with your friends, swim, take the stairs, or walk to the grocery store or work.

Combined, these habits may be a safe, healthy way to lose weight and keep it off.

Fact: Fad diets are not the best way to lose weight and keep it off. These diets often promise quick weight loss if you strictly reduce what you eat or avoid some types of foods. Some of these diets may help you lose weight at first. But these diets are hard to follow. Most people quickly get tired of them and regain any lost weight.

Fad diets may be unhealthy. They may not provide all of the nutrients your body needs. Also, losing more than 3 pounds a week after the first few weeks may increase your chances of developing gallstones (solid matter in the gallbladder that can cause pain). Being on a diet of fewer than 800 calories a day for a long time may lead to serious heart problems.

TIP: Research suggests that safe weight loss involves combining a reduced-calorie diet with physical activity to lose 1/2 to 2 pounds a week (after the first few weeks of weight loss). Make healthy food choices. Eat small portions. Build exercise into your daily life. Combined, these habits may be a healthy way to lose weight and keep it off. These habits may also lower your chances of developing heart disease, high blood pressure, and type 2 diabetes.

Myth: Grain products such as bread, pasta, and rice are

fattening. I should avoid them when trying to lose weight.

Fact: A grain product is any food made from wheat, rice, oats, cornmeal, barley, or another cereal grain. Grains are divided into two subgroups, whole grains and refined grains. Whole grains contain the entire grain kernel—the bran, germ, and endosperm. Examples include brown rice and whole-wheat bread, cereal, and pasta. Refined grains have been milled, a process that removes the bran and germ. This is done to give grains a finer texture and improve their shelf life, but it also removes dietary fiber, iron, and many B vitamins.

People who eat whole grains as part of a healthy diet may lower their chances of developing some chronic diseases. Government dietary guidelines advise making half your grains whole grains. For example, choose 100 percent whole-wheat bread instead of white bread, and brown rice instead of white rice.

TIP: To lose weight, reduce the number of calories you take in and increase the amount of physical activity you do each day. Create and follow a healthy eating plan that replaces less healthy options with a mix of fruits, veggies, whole grains, protein foods, and low-fat dairy:

Eat a mix of fat-free or low-fat milk and milk products, fruits, veggies, and whole grains.

Limit added sugars, cholesterol, salt (sodium), and saturated fat.

Eat low-fat protein: beans, eggs, fish, lean meats, nuts, and poultry.

Meal Myths

Myth: Some people can eat whatever they want and still lose weight.

Fact: To lose weight, you need to burn more calories than you eat and drink. Some people may seem to get away with eating any kind of food they want and still lose weight. But those people, like everyone, must use more energy than they take in through food and drink to lose weight.

A number of factors such as your age, genes, medicines, and lifestyle habits may affect your weight.

Eat the rainbow!

When making half of your plate fruits and veggies, choose foods with vibrant colors that are packed with fiber, minerals, and vitamins.

Red: bell peppers, cherries, cranberries, onions, red beets, strawberries, tomatoes, watermelon.

Green: avocado, broccoli, cabbage, cucumber, dark lettuce, grapes, honeydew, kale, kiwi, spinach, zucchini.

Orange and yellow: apricots, bananas, carrots, mangoes, oranges, peaches, squash, sweet potatoes.

Blue and purple: blackberries, blueberries, grapes, plums, purple cabbage, purple carrots, purple potatoes.

TIP: When trying to lose weight, you can still eat your favorite foods as part of a healthy eating plan. But you must watch the total number of calories that you eat. Reduce your portion sizes (see below to understand portions and servings). Find ways to limit the calories in your favorite foods. For example, you can bake foods rather than frying them. Use low-fat milk in place of cream. Make half of your plate fruits and veggies.

Myth: "Low-fat" or "fat-free" means no calories.

Fact: A serving of low-fat or fat-free food may be lower in calories than a serving of the full-fat product. But many processed low-fat or fat-free foods have just as many calories as the full-fat versions of the same foods—or even more calories. These foods may contain added flour, salt, starch, or sugar to improve flavor and texture after fat is removed. These items add calories.

What is the difference between a serving and a portion?

The U.S. Food and Drug Administration (FDA) Nutrition Facts label appears on most packaged foods. It tells you how many calories and servings are in a box or can. The serving size varies from product to product.

A portion is how much food you choose to eat at one time, whether in a restaurant, from a package, or at home. Sometimes the serving size and portion size match; sometimes they do not.

You can use the Nutrition Facts label

to track your calorie intake and number of servings

to make healthy food choices by serving smaller portions and selecting items lower in fats, salt, and sugar and higher in fiber and vitamins

TIP: Read the Nutrition Facts label on a food package to find out how many calories are in a serving. Check the serving size, too—it may be less than you are used to eating.

Myth: Fast foods are always an unhealthy choice. You should not eat them when dieting.

Fact: Many fast foods are unhealthy and may affect weight gain. However, if you do eat fast food, choose menu options with care. Both at home and away, choose healthy foods that are nutrient rich, low in calories, and small in portion size.

TIP: To choose healthy, low-calorie options, check the nutrition facts. These are often offered on the menu or on restaurant websites. And know that the nutrition facts often do not include sauces and extras. Try these tips:

Avoid "value" combo meals, which tend to have more calories than you need in one meal.

Choose fresh fruit items or nonfat yogurt for dessert.

Limit your use of toppings that are high in fat and

calories, such as bacon, cheese, regular mayonnaise, salad dressings, and tartar sauce.

Pick steamed or baked items over fried ones.

Sip on water or fat-free milk instead of soda.

Myth: If I skip meals, I can lose weight.

Fact: Skipping meals may make you feel hungrier and lead you to eat more than you normally would at your next meal. In particular, studies show a link between skipping breakfast and obesity. People who skip breakfast tend to be heavier than people who eat a healthy breakfast.

TIP: Choose meals and snacks that include a variety of healthy foods. Try these examples:

For a quick breakfast, make oatmeal with low-fat milk, topped with fresh berries. Or eat a slice of whole-wheat toast with fruit spread.

Pack a healthy lunch each night, so you won't be tempted to rush out of the house in the morning without one.

For healthy nibbles, pack a small low-fat yogurt, a couple of whole-wheat crackers with peanut butter, or veggies with hummus.

Fact: Eating better does not have to cost a lot of money. Many people think that fresh foods are healthier than canned or frozen ones. For example, some people think that spinach is better for you raw than frozen or canned. However, canned or frozen fruits and veggies provide as many nutrients as fresh ones, at a lower cost. Healthy options include low-salt canned veggies and fruit canned in its own juice or water-packed. Remember to rinse canned veggies to remove excess salt. Also, some canned seafood, like tuna, is easy to keep on the shelf, healthy, and low-cost. And canned, dried, or frozen beans, lentils, and peas are also healthy sources of protein that are easy on the wallet.

TIP: Check the nutrition facts on canned, dried, and frozen items. Look for items that are high in calcium, fiber, potassium, protein, and vitamin D. Also check for items that are low in added sugars, saturated fat, and sodium.

Physical Activity Myths

Don't just sit there!

Americans spend a lot of time sitting in front of computers, desks, hand-held devices, and TVs. Break up your day by moving around more and getting regular aerobic activity that makes you sweat and breathe faster.

Get 150 to 300 minutes of moderately intense or vigorous physical activity each week. Basketball, brisk walks, hikes, hula hoops, runs, soccer, tennis—choose whatever you enjoy best! Even 10 minutes of activity at a time can add up over the week.

Strengthen your muscles at least twice a week. Do push-ups or pull-ups, lift weights, do heavy gardening, or work with rubber resistance bands.

Myth: Lifting weights is not a good way to lose weight because it will make me "bulk up."

Fact: Lifting weights or doing activities like push-ups and crunches on a regular basis can help you build strong muscles, which can help you burn more calories. To strengthen muscles, you can lift weights, use large rubber bands (resistance bands), do push-ups or sit-ups, or do household or yard tasks that make you lift or dig. Doing strengthening activities 2 or 3 days a week will not "bulk you up." Only intense strength training, along with certain genetics, can build large muscles.

TIP: Government guidelines for physical activity recommend that adults should do activities at least two times a week to strengthen muscles. The guidelines also suggest that adults should get 150 to 300 minutes of moderately intense or vigorous aerobic activity each week—like brisk walking or biking. Aerobic activity makes you sweat and breathe faster.

Myth: Physical activity only counts if I can do it for long periods of time.

Fact: You do not need to be active for long periods to achieve your 150 to 300 minutes of activity each week. Experts advise doing aerobic activity for periods of 10 minutes or longer at a time. You can spread these sessions out over the week.

TIP: Plan to do at least 10 minutes of physical activity three times a day on 5 or more days a week. This will help you meet the 150-minute goal. While at work, take a brief walking break. Use the stairs. Get off the bus one stop early. Go dancing with friends. Whether for a short or long period, bursts of activity may add up to the total amount of physical activity you need each week.

Food Myths

Myth: Eating meat is bad for my health and makes it harder to lose weight.

Fact: Eating lean meat in small amounts can be part of a healthy plan to lose weight. Chicken, fish, pork, and red meat contain some cholesterol and saturated fat. But they also contain healthy nutrients like iron, protein, and zinc.

TIP: Choose cuts of meat that are lower in fat, and trim off all the fat you can see. Meats that are lower in fat include chicken breast, pork loin and beef round steak, flank steak, and extra lean ground beef. Also, watch portion size. Try to eat meat or poultry in portions of 3 ounces or less. Three ounces is about the size of a deck of cards.

Myth: Dairy products are fattening and unhealthy.

Fact: Fat-free and low-fat cheese, milk, and yogurt are just as healthy as whole-milk dairy products, and they are lower in fat and calories. Dairy products offer protein to build muscles and help organs work well, and calcium to strengthen bones. Most milk and some yogurts have extra vitamin D added to help your body use calcium. Most Americans don't get enough calcium and vitamin D. Dairy is an easy way to get more of these nutrients.

TIP: Based on Government guidelines, you should try to have 3 cups a day of fat-free or low-fat milk or milk products. This can include soy beverages fortified with vitamins. If you can't digest lactose (the sugar found in dairy products), choose lactose-free or low-lactose dairy products or other foods and beverages that have calcium and vitamin D:

calcium: soy-based beverages or tofu made with calcium sulfate; canned salmon; dark leafy greens like collards or kale

vitamin D: cereals or soy-based beverages

Myth: "Going vegetarian" will help me lose weight and be healthier.

Fact: Research shows that people who follow a vegetarian eating plan, on average, eat fewer calories and less fat than non-vegetarians. Some research has found that vegetarian-style eating patterns are associated with lower levels of obesity, lower blood pressure, and a reduced risk of heart disease.

Vegetarians also tend to have lower body mass index (BMI) scores than people with other eating plans. (The BMI measures body fat based on a person's height in relation to weight). But vegetarians—like others—can make food choices that impact weight gain, like eating large amounts of foods that are high in fat or calories or low in nutrients.

The types of vegetarian diets eaten in the United States can vary widely. Vegans do not consume any animal products, while lacto-ovo vegetarians eat milk and eggs along with plant foods. Some people have eating patterns that are mainly vegetarian but may include small amounts of meat, poultry, or seafood.

TIP: If you choose to follow a vegetarian eating plan, be sure you get enough of the nutrients that others usually take in from animal products such as cheese, eggs, meat, and milk. Nutrients that may be lacking in a vegetarian diet are listed below, along with foods and beverages that may help you meet your body's needs for these nutrients.

Nutrient - Common Sources

Calcium - dairy products, soy beverages with added calcium, tofu made with calcium sulfate, collard greens, kale, broccoli.

Iron - cashews, spinach, lentils, chickpeas, bread or cereal with added iron.

Protein - eggs, dairy products, beans, peas, nuts, seeds, tofu, tempeh, soy-based burgers.

Vitamin B12 - eggs, dairy products, fortified cereal or soy beverages, tempeh, miso (tempeh and miso are foods made from soybeans).

Vitamin D - foods and beverages with added vitamin D, including milk, soy beverages, or cereal.

Zinc - whole grains (check the ingredients list on product labels for the words "whole" or "whole grain" before the grain ingredient's name), nuts, tofu, leafy greens (spinach, cabbage, lettuce).

22. Ten Great Ideas to Boost Your Weight Loss Efforts

Sometimes we need rules and guidelines to follow, it makes things easier for us. With that in mind, I hereby announce the 10 Commandments Of Weight Loss!

1. Lifestyle, Not a Diet

This is not a short term fix; it's a way of life. Treat it as such and you will definitely see the results you want.

2. Get Organized

Structure your life and you'll structure your eating. There are tons of meal plans out there that can help bring you more structure.

3. Eat Small

Portion control is crucial for losing weight. You'll learn that it is not necessary to "clean your plate" every time. Pay attention to the portion sizes that your meal plan recommends.

4. Learn to Leave Food on Your Plate

This helps you take control of compulsive eating. Once you start feeling more in control of your impulses, the better you feel about yourself.

5. Never Feel Deprived

This only encourages binging. Try to eat small portions all day, so you feel full.

6. Make a Meal Out of It

Make a ceremony out of every meal, so that you really appreciate what you've eaten. It doesn't take much. You can light candles, set the table, adopt a meal-preparing habit, whatever works for you.

7. Eat Slowly

That way, you'll feel satisfied before you've eaten too much.

8. Enjoy Your Food

It's one of life's greatest pleasures, not a punishment. Appreciate the tastes, colors, textures of your food. Take the time to think about how much effort has gone into creating what's on your plate. From the time it takes to grow your food, to the logistical process of how it gets to your plate. The fact is, what you eat is what gives your body the materials it needs to keep going. So give it great materials!

9. Move It!

Exercise is an essential part of losing weight. Plus it releases endorphins into your bloodstream and makes you feel great!

10. Get Enough Sleep

Who couldn't be OK with this one? Structuring your sleeping patterns will not only make you more enjoyable to be around, it will regulate your metabolism.

23. Don't Read This If You Want To Remain Overweight For The Rest of Your Life

Here Are Some Important Weight Loss Facts You Need to Know:

Weight loss can be achieved either by eating fewer calories or by burning more calories with physical activity, preferably both.

A healthy weight loss program consists of:

A reasonable, realistic weight loss goal

A reduced calorie, nutritionally-balanced eating plan

Regular physical activity

A behavior change plan to help you stay on track with your goals

You need to consider each of these components.

Keep in Mind

Calories count

Portions count

Nutrition counts

Even a small amount of weight loss can lead to big health benefits

Strive to develop good habits to last a lifetime

Discuss weight loss with your doctor before getting started

Getting Started

Check your Body Mass Index (BMI) - an indicator of body fat - and see where it fits within the BMI categories.

Discuss weight loss with your doctor and decide on a goal. If you have a lot of weight to lose, set a realistic intermediate goal, maybe to lose 10 pounds. Remember that even a small amount of weight loss can lead to big health benefits.

Estimate your calorie needs. Using this tool, you can determine the number of calories needed each day to maintain your current weight. To lose about 1 pound per week, subtract 500 calories each day from the daily amount. To lose about 2 pounds per week, subtract 1000 calories daily.

Score your current food intake and physical activity level. Taking a good look at your current habits will help you determine what changes you might make as well as what you are doing right.

How Do I Know Which Weight Loss Plan is Right For Me?

Keep in mind that you want to develop lifestyle habits that will help you maintain your weight in a healthy range. A short-term "diet" that you "go on" and then "go off" is not the answer to long-term weight management.

In choosing how to go about losing weight, keep in mind key habits of people who have lost weight and kept in off. These people are called "Successful Losers" by the weight control experts who have studied them.

Key Behaviors of Successful Losers

Getting regular physical activity

Reducing calorie and fat intake

Eating regular meals, including breakfast

Weighing themselves regularly

Not letting small "slips" turn into large weight regain

Staying On Track with Your Goals

Setting realistic goals and tracking your progress are key to your success. In fact, research has shown that those who keep track of their behaviors are more likely to take off weight and keep it off. A reasonable rate of weight loss is 1 to 2 pounds per week.

24. Everything You Always Wanted to Know About Weight Loss But Were Afraid to Ask

(This chapter is based on info provided by the US government)

How do I know if I'm overweight or obese?

Body Mass Index

You can find out your BMI by using this calculator. Find out your body mass index (BMI). BMI is a measure of body fat based on height and weight. People with a BMI of 25 to 29.9 are considered overweight. People with a BMI of 30 or more are considered obese.

What causes someone to become overweight or obese?

You can become overweight or obese when you eat more calories than you use. A calorie is a unit of energy in the food you eat. Your body needs this energy to function and to be active. But if you take in more energy than your body uses, you will gain weight.

Many factors can play a role in becoming overweight or obese. These factors include:

Behaviors, such as eating too many calories or not getting enough physical activity

Environment and culture

Genes

Overweight and obesity problems keep getting worse in the United States. Some cultural reasons for this include:

Bigger portion sizes

Little time to exercise or cook healthy meals

Using cars to get places instead of walking

What are the health effects of being overweight or obese?

Being overweight or obese can increase your risk of:

Heart disease

Stroke

Type 2 diabetes

High blood pressure

Breathing problems

Arthritis

Gallbladder disease

Some kinds of cancer

But excess body weight isn't the only health risk. The places where you store your body fat also affect your health. Women with a "pear" shape tend to store fat in their hips and buttocks. Women with an "apple" shape store fat around their waists. If your waist is more than 35 inches, you may have a higher risk of weight-related health problems.

What is the best way for me to lose weight?

The best way to lose weight is to use more calories than you take in. You can do this by following a healthy eating plan and being more active. Before you start a weight-loss program, talk to your doctor.

Safe weight-loss programs that work well:

Set a goal of slow and steady weight loss — 1 to 2 pounds per week

Offer low-calorie eating plans with a wide range of healthy foods

Encourage you to be more physically active

Teach you about healthy eating and physical activity

Adapt to your likes and dislikes and cultural background

Help you keep weight off after you lose it

How can I make healthier food choices?

Focus on fruits. Eat a variety of fruits — fresh, frozen, canned, or dried — rather than fruit juice for most of your fruit choices. For a 2,000-calorie diet, you will need 2 cups of fruit each day. An example of 2 cups is 1 small banana, 1 large orange, and 1/4 cup of dried apricots or peaches.

Vary your veggies. Eat more:

dark green veggies, such as broccoli, kale, and other dark leafy greens

orange veggies, such as carrots, sweet potatoes, pumpkin, and winter squash

beans and peas, such as pinto beans, kidney beans, black beans, garbanzo beans, split peas, and lentils

Get your calcium-rich foods. Each day, drink 3 cups of low-fat or fat-free milk. Or, you can get an equivalent amount of low-fat yogurt and/or low-fat cheese each day. 1.5 ounces of cheese equals 1 cup of milk. If you don't or can't consume milk, choose lactose-free milk products and/or calcium-fortified foods and drinks.

Make half your grains whole. Eat at least 3 ounces of whole-grain cereals, breads, crackers, rice, or pasta each day. One ounce is about 1 slice of bread, 1 cup of breakfast cereal, or 1/2 cup of cooked rice or pasta. Look to see that grains such as wheat, rice, oats, or corn are referred to as "whole" in the list of ingredients.

Go lean with protein. Choose lean meats and poultry. Bake it, broil it, or grill it. Vary your protein choices with more fish, beans, peas, nuts, and seeds.

Limit saturated fats. Get less than 10 percent of your calories from saturated fatty acids. Most fats should come from sources of polyunsaturated and mono-unsaturated fatty acids, such as fish, nuts, and vegetable oils. When choosing and preparing meat, poultry, dry beans, and milk or milk products, make choices that are lean, low-fat, or fat-free.

Limit salt. Get less than 2,300 mg of sodium (about 1 teaspoon of salt) each day.

An active lifestyle can lower your risk of early death from a variety of causes. There is strong evidence that regular physical activity can also lower your risk of:

Heart disease

Stroke

High blood pressure

Unhealthy cholesterol levels

Type 2 diabetes

Metabolic syndrome

Colon cancer

Breast cancer

Falls

Depression

Regular activity can help prevent unhealthy weight gain and also help with weight loss, when combined with lower calorie intake. If you are overweight or obese, losing weight can lower your risk for many diseases. Being overweight or obese increases your risk of heart disease, high blood pressure, stroke, type 2 diabetes, breathing problems, osteoarthritis, gallbladder disease, sleep apnea (breathing problems while sleeping), and some cancers.

Regular physical activity can also improve your cardiorespiratory (heart, lungs, and blood vessels) and muscular fitness. For older adults, activity can improve mental function.

Physical activity may also help:

Improve functional health for older adults

Reduce waistline size

Lower risk of hip fracture

Lower risk of lung cancer

Lower risk of endometrial cancer

Maintain weight after weight loss

Increase bone density

Improve sleep quality

Health benefits are gained by doing the following each week:

Moderate activity

During moderate-intensity activities you should notice an increase in your heart rate, but you should still be able to talk comfortably. An example of a moderate-intensity activity is walking on a level surface at a brisk pace (about 3 to 4 miles per hour). Other examples include ballroom dancing, leisurely bicycling, moderate housework, and waiting tables.

Vigorous activity

If your heart rate increases a lot and you are breathing so hard that it is difficult to carry on a conversation, you are probably doing vigorous-intensity activity. Examples of vigorous-intensity activities include jogging, bicycling fast or uphill, singles tennis, and pushing a hand mower.

2 hours and 30 minutes of moderate-intensity aerobic physical activity

or

1 hour and 15 minutes of vigorous-intensity aerobic physical activity

or

A combination of moderate and vigorous-intensity aerobic physical activity

and

Muscle-strengthening activities on 2 or more days

This physical activity should be in addition to your routine activities of daily living, such as cleaning or spending a few minutes walking from the parking lot to your office.

If you want to lose a substantial (more than 5 percent of body weight) amount of weight, you need a high amount of physical activity unless you also lower calorie intake. This is also the case if you are trying to keep the weight off. Many people need to do more than 300 minutes of moderate-intensity activity a week to meet weight-control goals.

What medicines are approved for long-term treatment of obesity?

The Food and Drug Administration has approved two medicines for long-term treatment of obesity:

Sibutramine (si-BYOO-tra-meen) suppresses your appetite.

Orlistat (OR-li-stat) keeps your body from absorbing fat from the food you eat.

These medicines are for people who:

Have a BMI of 30 or higher

Have a BMI of 27 or higher and weight-related health problems or health risks

If you take these medicines, you will need to follow a healthy eating and physical activity plan at the same time.

Before taking these medicines, talk with your doctor about the benefits and the side effects.

Sibutramine can raise your blood pressure and heart rate. You should not take this medicine if you have a history of high blood pressure, heart problems, or strokes. Other side effects include dry mouth, headache, constipation, anxiety, and trouble sleeping.

Orlistat may cause diarrhea, cramping, gas, and leakage of oily stool. Eating a low-fat diet can help prevent these side effects. This medicine may also prevent your body from absorbing some vitamins. Talk with your doctor about whether you should take a vitamin supplement.

What surgical options are used to treat obesity?

Weight loss surgeries — also called bariatric (bair-ee-AT-rik) surgeries — can help treat obesity. You should only consider surgical treatment for weight loss if you:

Have a BMI of 40 or higher

Have a BMI of 35 or higher and weight-related health problems

Have not had success with other weight-loss methods

Common types of weight loss surgeries are:

Roux-en-Y (ROO-en-WEYE) gastric bypass. The surgeon uses surgical staples to create a small stomach pouch. This limits the amount of food you can eat. The pouch is attached to the middle part of the small intestine. Food bypasses the upper part of the small intestine and stomach, reducing the amount of calories and nutrients your body absorbs.

Laparoscopic (LAP-uh-ruh-SKAWP-ik) gastric banding. A band is placed around the upper stomach to create a small pouch and narrow passage into the rest of the stomach. This limits the amount of food you can eat. The size of the band can be adjusted. A surgeon can remove the band if needed.

Biliopancreatic (bil-ee-oh-pan-kree-at-ik) diversion (BPD) or BPD with duodenal (doo-AW-duh-nul) switch (BPD/DS). In BPD, a large part of the stomach is removed, leaving a small pouch. The pouch is connected to the last part of the small intestine, bypassing other parts of the small intestine. In BPD/DS, less of the stomach and small intestine are removed. This surgery reduces the amount of food you can eat and the amount of calories and nutrients your body absorbs from food. This surgery is used less often than other types of surgery because of the high risk of malnutrition.

If you are thinking about weight-loss surgery, talk with your doctor about changes you will need to make after the surgery. You will need to:

Follow your doctor's directions as you heal

Make lasting changes in the way you eat

Follow a healthy eating plan and be physically active

Take vitamins and minerals if needed

You should also talk to your doctor about risks and side effects of weight loss surgery. Side effects may include:

Infection

Leaking from staples

Hernia

Blood clots in the leg veins that travel to your lungs (pulmonary embolism)

Dumping syndrome, in which food moves from your stomach to your intestines too quickly

Not getting enough vitamins and minerals from food

Is liposuction a treatment for obesity?

Liposuction (LY-poh-suhk-shuhn) is not a treatment for obesity. In this procedure, a surgeon removes fat from under the skin. Liposuction can be used to reshape parts of your body. But this surgery does not promise lasting weight loss.

I'm concerned about my children's eating and physical activity levels. How can I help improve their habits?

The things children learn when they are young are hard to change as they get older. This is true for their eating and physical activity habits. Many children have a poor diet and are not very active. They may eat foods high in calories and fat and not eat enough fruits and vegetables. They also may watch TV, play video games, or use the computer instead of being active.

Kids who are overweight have a greater chance of becoming obese adults. Overweight children may develop weight-related health problems like high blood pressure and diabetes at a young age. You can find out if your child is overweight or obese by using the Body Mass Index for children and teens.

Body Mass Index for children and teens

You can find out your child's BMI by using the calculator at girlshealth.gov

You can help your child build healthy eating and activity habits.

Limit time spent watching TV, playing video games, and using the computer.

Make sure your child is physically active for 1 hour each day.

Find out about activity programs in your community.

Ask your children what they like to do and what they'd like to try, like Little League Baseball or a swim team.

Plan activities for the whole family — like hiking, walking, or playing ball.

Help your children eat healthy foods.

Have your children plan and cook healthy meals with you.

Don't do other things while you eat, like watch TV.

Give your kids healthy snacks, like fruits, whole-grain crackers, and vegetables.

Limit your trips to fast-food restaurants.

Involve the whole family in healthy eating. Don't single out your children by their weight.

We know children do what they see — not always what they are told. Set a good example for your children. Your kids will learn to eat right and be active by watching you. Setting a good example can mean a lifetime of good habits for you and your kids.

25. The Culprit of Your Overweight Problems Has Been Finally Identified (Humor)

Ever wonder who is to blame for your weight loss suffering? Well, wonder no more. Here's the full story.

And God populated the earth with broccoli and cauliflower and spinach, green and yellow vegetables of all kinds, so Man and Woman would live long and healthy lives.

And Satan created McDonald's. And McDonald's brought forth the 99-cent double-cheeseburger. And Satan said to Man, "You want fries with that?"

And Man said, "Super size them."

And Man gained pounds.

And God created the healthful yogurt, that woman might keep her figure that man found so fair.

And Satan brought forth chocolate.

And woman gained pounds.

And God said, "Try my crispy fresh salad."

And Satan brought forth ice cream.

And woman gained pounds. And God said, "I have sent you heart healthy vegetables and olive oil with which to cook them."

And Satan brought forth chicken-fried steak so big it needed its own platter.

And Man gained pounds and his bad cholesterol went through the roof.

And God brought forth running shoes and Man resolved to lose those extra pounds.

And Satan brought forth cable TV with remote control so Man would not have to toil to change channels between ESPN and ESPN2.

And Man gained pounds.

And God said, "You're running up the score, Devil."

And God brought forth the potato, a vegetable naturally low in fat and brimming with nutrition.

And Satan peeled off the healthful skin and sliced the starchy center into chips and deep-fat fried them. And he created sour cream dip also.

And Man clutched his remote control and ate the potato chips swaddled in cholesterol.

And Satan saw and said, "It is good."

And Man went into cardiac arrest.

And God sighed and created quadruple bypass surgery.

And so, Satan created HMOs.

26. Fear And Loathing in The Gym (Humor)

Dear Diary,

For my 50th birthday, my husband, the dear, purchased a week of personal training at the local health club for me.

Although I am still in great shape since playing on my high school softball team, I decided it would be a good idea to go ahead and give it a try.

I called the club and made my reservations with a personal trainer I'll call Bruce, who identified himself as a 26 year old aerobics instructor and model for athletic clothing and swim wear.

My husband seemed pleased with my enthusiasm to get started. The club encouraged me to keep this diary to chart my progress...

Monday: Started my day at 6:00 a.m. Tough to get out of bed, but found it was well worth the effort when I arrived at the health club and found Bruce waiting for me. He is something of a Greek God! with blonde hair, dancing blue eyes and a dazzling white smile. Woo Hoo!!!

Bruce gave me a tour and showed me the machines. He took my pulse after five minutes on the treadmill. He was alarmed that my pulse was so fast, but I attribute it to standing next to him in his Lycra aerobic outfit. I enjoyed watching the skillful way in which he conducted his aerobics class after my workout today. Very inspiring!

Bruce was encouraging as I did my sit-ups, although my gut was already aching from holding it in the whole time he was around. This is going to be a FANTASTIC week!

Tuesday: I drank a whole pot of coffee, but I finally made it out the door. Bruce made me lie on my back and push a heavy iron bar into the air, then he put weights on it! My legs were a little wobbly on the treadmill, but I made the full mile. Bruce's rewarding smile made it all worthwhile. I feel GREAT!! It's a whole new life for me!!!

Wednesday: The only way I can brush my teeth is by laying on the toothbrush on the counter and moving my mouth back and forth over it. I believe I have a hernia in both pectorals. Driving was OK as long as I didn't try to steer or to stop. I parked on top of a GEO in the club parking lot. Bruce was impatient with me, insisting that my screams bothered the other club members. His voice is a little too perky for early in the morning and when he scolds he gets this nasally whine that is VERY annoying. My chest hurt when I got on the treadmill, so Bruce put me on the stair monster. Why the heck would anyone invent a machine to simulate an activity rendered obsolete by elevators? Bruce told me it would help me get in shape and enjoy life. He said some other useless sh** too!

Thursday: Bruce was waiting for me with his vampire-like teeth exposed as his thin, cruel lips were pulled back in a full snarl. I couldn't help being half an hour late, it took me that long to tie my shoes! Bruce took me to work out with dumbbells. When he was not looking, I ran and hid in the men's room. He sent Lars in to find me, then, as punishment, put me on the rowing machine, which I promptly sank!

Friday: I hate that son-of-a b**** Bruce more than any human being has ever hated any other human being in the history of the world. Stupid, skinny, anemic little cheerleader wanna-be! If there was a part of my body I could move without unbearable pain, I would beat him with it! Bruce wanted me to work on my triceps. I don't have any triceps!!! And if you don't want dents in the floor don't hand me the %&$#&%&# barbells or anything that weighs more than a sandwich! (which I am sure you learned in the sadist school you attended and graduated magna cum laude!)

The treadmill flung me off and I landed on a health and nutrition teacher. Why couldn't it have been someone softer, like the drama coach of the choir director?

Saturday: Bruce left a message on my answering machine in his grating, shrill voice wondering why I did not show up today. Just hearing him made me want to smash the machine with my planner. However, I lacked the strength to even use the TV remote and ended up catching eleven straight hours of the *&$%^$& weather channel!!!

Sunday: I'm having the Church van pick me up for services

today so I can go and thank God that this week is over. I will also pray that next year my husband will choose a gift for me that is fun---- like a root canal or hysterectomy.

Beyond Dieting

Take time to laugh
It is the music of the soul.

Take time to think
It is the source of power.

Take time to play
It is the source of perpetual youth.

Take time to read
It is the fountain of wisdom.

Take time to pray
It is the greatest power on earth.

Take time to love and be loved
It is a God-given privilege.

Take time to be friendly
It is the road to happiness.

Take time to give
It is too short a day to be selfish.

Take time to work
It is the price of success.

DR. ADAM COLTON